FAT-BURNING FEAST

FAT-BURNING FEAST

Keto Meals for Optimal Weight Loss

JULES HAWTHORNE

QuillQuest Publishers

CONTENTS

1	Introduction	1
2	Benefits of a Keto Diet	3
3	Getting Started with Keto	5
4	Planning Your Meals	7
5	Breakfast Recipes	9
6	Lunch Recipes	11
7	Dinner Recipes	13
8	Snack Ideas	16
9	Dessert Options	17
10	Beverages to Aid Weight Loss	19
11	Tips for Successful Weight Loss	21
12	Exercise and Keto Diet	23
13	Tracking Your Progress	25
14	Overcoming Challenges	27
15	Frequently Asked Questions	29
16	Conclusion	31

Copyright © 2024 by Jules Hawthorne

All rights reserved. No part of this book may be reproduced in any manner whatsoever without written permission except in the case of brief quotations embodied in critical articles and reviews.

First Printing, 2024

CHAPTER 1

Introduction

The recipes here are organized in a way that makes it easy for you to figure out exactly what to eat for breakfast, lunch, and dinner, plus it simplifies things come snack time. The recipes in this book are strategically Goldilocks' style – they are not hard or complicated; they are just right! And most important, you'll love that all the meals in this book are keto – all 30 are specifically designed to keep your body in fat-burning mode. This is the first recipe you see when you flip through this book. I placed this right up front to tell you that it is utterly delicious and the taste, awesomeness-level high! When you really can't figure out what to make but you want something that's going to be delicious and convenient to eat, choose this. You'll be jumping for joy the moment you chow down, knowing this whole spread is keto-perfect for your health and weight-loss goals.

Are you looking for tasty, mouthwatering and simple keto recipes to help you burn fat optimally? Do you think losing weight on keto means you have to spend hours in the kitchen? Just because you're eating low-carb doesn't mean you've got to resort to hamburger patties and salad for every meal. No way! There are 30 quick and easy recipes in this book committed to burning fat for you with uninterrupted and efficient weight loss. No matter what your taste buds desire, you'll find something to whet your taste buds that won't increase your pant size. You'll love knowing that your meals are all keto, relative to your ultimate weight loss goals. Plus, this keto feast is uncomplicated and smart, just like you!

CHAPTER 2

Benefits of a Keto Diet

The true benefit of fat metabolism occurs when ketones are produced in very high numbers - this state is called nutritional ketosis. An efficient fat burn starts when blood ketone levels move above 0.5 mmol/l (millimoles per litre). This is the ideal mark if the ultimate goal is improving overall health, losing weight and safeguarding the brain. Any diet that manages to keep this stage going consistently is considered successful in aiding the body's weight loss efforts. In addition, dramatic increase in the number of ketones in the blood results in a near absence of hunger, decreased cravings and improved mental clarity. Maintaining nutritional ketosis for an extended period of time can also provide a sense of calmness and consistent energy, as well as help prevent a number of chronic diseases associated with poor nutrition, such as Type 2 diabetes, metabolic syndrome, neurodegenerative diseases and some types of cancer.

Introduction: Ketosis or 'fat-burning' is one of the most efficient and safe ways to lose weight. It has been used (and studied) for over a hundred years. Ketosis is a completely natural metabolic state that occurs as a result of our body's inability to use up all carbohydrates that are consumed. When the carbohydrate intake is restricted, the body begins to break down stored fats and uses fatty acids (from stored body fat or dietary fat) to fuel itself. The byproducts of fat breakdown are ketone bodies that replace glucose as the primary source of body fuel. All the cells and organs can use ketones for energy but the brain is particularly happy on this kind of 'clean' fuel, as its main function is providing power to the rest of the body. When the body runs on ketones, blood sugar levels and insulin resistance improve - two factors that are often responsible for excessive weight gain and inability to lose weight.

CHAPTER 3

Getting Started with Keto

By this time, your body has already experienced withdrawing from sugar. Missing your favorite treats, and has begun to become fat adapted. Now you can adapt to the next phase of your diet regiment. No veggies at this time, now you are consuming fats, moderate proteins, and cerebous grains. Getting ready to eliminate all grains, the first three days of week 3 will be the worse time. It is during the first 3 days of the week when you will feel the true effects of keto. You will feel drained, weak, and non-energetic. Your skin may become an oil field, and your hair may look greasy and unwashed. You may feel like taking the day off from work or school and your joints will start to feel achy. Remember, this is the time when you detox. It's also the time your body makes the keto adjustment! The complete withdrawal of grains, including cerebous grains, will have a tremendous impact on your digestive system and organs. The low carb diet allows the micro-villi in your digestive system to grow and fully develop. This will enable your bacteria to properly function better healing your organs, tissue, and skin conditions. The important thing is to keep sugar intake low. Eliminate grains from the first three days this week, and use fats for energy. This is the time to drink bone broths, and eat sardine/grainy/oily fish.

    The ketogenic diet emphasizes high fat, moderate protein, and very low carbohydrate consumption. Hold up—fat? Isn't that the stuff that causes heart disease and makes you gain weight? Not exactly. In fact, fats can make your body more efficient at burning fat. The 1st week on keto can throw you some curve balls that can put some off. To make it easier for you, ease your way into it. Here are a few things that you can do to make adjusting to a keto diet more doable. Break the diet into two parts. Get started this first week by eating all the veggies and fruits you want, including refined food products such as pasta made with flour and flavors. In other words, eat healthily. The start of week 2 is the time to break sugar, wheat and refined flour addiction. At this point, all refined foods will be out of your system and good to go.

CHAPTER 4

Planning Your Meals

In other words, on Keto, you can eat food just like everyone else. With Keto, the only thing you need to think about is what to eat with your food! So whether you pick out a skinless, boneless chicken breast for dinner, or pick out an extra-fatty steak, you'll be able to have your choice of vegetables and salad toppings plus a heart-healthy serving of healthful fats to go alongside it. And similarly, whether you pick out an extra-lean ground turkey for your salads all week long, or you stock the fridge with thick, juicy 80/20 beef patties, you'll be able to pair your meat with good-for-you veggies and quality fats. Once you have a deep enough understanding of healthful fats and how to prepare nutrient-rich meals, I believe that traveling the path of faith is enough to fulfill all your Keto-meal planning precepts.

At this point, you know enough about the Keto diet to know that when you eat Keto, you need to make sure you include a source of healthy fats in every meal. Most people are surprised to realize that planning a Keto meal is actually very straightforward, sometimes even easier than planning a meal on other diets. If you were to have a meal on a typical low-fat diet, there are a number of different food items that "count" as a serving of protein food, for example. People on a low-fat diet are usually required to plan a meal with only a certain amount of vegetables, a certain amount of whole grains (or fruit), and a very small serving of heart-healthy fat. With Keto, though, things are really quite a bit more straightforward: you just need to make sure you make a meal that includes a source of healthy fats.

CHAPTER 5

Breakfast Recipes

For good or evil, you're getting those clean, high-fat calories with bulletproof coffee, which is just coffee with grass-fed butter or coconut oil. We like grass-fed butter; the creaminess is hard to beat and there's no risk of the coconut oil curdling. (For that reason, you might consider starting with half the coconut oil and working your way up to a whole tablespoon.) Still, it's not a great idea to stir it up with a spoon and stubbornly refuse to consider a blender. Blenders and hand blenders emulsify everything, giving your coffee a great frothy head and ensuring there won't be a pool of oil on top. If you use a hand blender, I recommend adding the stevia before you blend in case more sweetness is necessary. More people are paying attention to this advice and realizing the benefits of the coffee than are noticing the connection between this coffee and the diet it was named after. For those unfamiliar with Bulletproof coffee and the Bulletproof diet, the primary point being made is that a combination of good fat right away in the morning is a great start to your day.

Hard-boiled eggs are a newborn ketogenic eater's best friend. A couple of those and some pork or turkey bacon are the perfect introduction to eating in the mornings without carbs. Here's another great breakfast meal prep: this recipe. Want to feel full all day on one hearty breakfast? This is it. Be sure to have grass-fed butter for making the Hollandaise sauce. You'll be on cloud nine all day after a breakfast like this - I promise.

CHAPTER 6

Lunch Recipes

Preheat the oven to 350°F (180°C). Line a 9 by 5-inch (23 by 13 cm) loaf pan with parchment paper. Add the beef, almond flour, Worcestershire sauce, egg, Dijon mustard, garlic, 1 tablespoon of the Italian seasoning, salt, and pepper to a large bowl. And add the parsley on top. Pour the tomato sauce over everything, and then cover with your hands to combine. Put the meat loaf mixture into the lined loaf pan, and form it into a loaf shape. Sprinkle the remaining 1 1/2 teaspoons of Italian seasoning over the top. Bake for 60 minutes. Remove the meat loaf from the oven, and let it sit uncovered for 5 minutes prior to slicing and serving. Serve the meat loaf with the stir-fried cabbage and the avocado wasabi cream for a delightful keto feast that is simple to prepare, and warming and satisfying to eat.

If you can give me the time to carefully review my options well ahead of time, making the right choices when it comes to feeding myself, most of the time, even if I am busy caring for others, is really not a problem. I have become the type of meal preparer who can get into the kitchen, pull out all the ingredients I need for the week's worth of meals, and speed through the process because I have become efficient in my daily and weekly food preparation efforts.

This particular meat loaf varies slightly from the traditional version, but slices and tastes like the original. It also helps me maintain my weight by keeping my carb count low, due to the substitutions of almond flour for bread crumbs, no-sugar-added tomato sauce for the typical ketchup ingredients, and other adaptations used to keep the carb count under 5 grams.

CHAPTER 7

Dinner Recipes

If you don't want to make barbecued salmon burgers with cucumber-avocado salad, we also offer a complete repertoire of other dinner recipes. Whichever you choose, you can expect your body to continue to burn fat and transition into deep sleep with comfort and ease. Until the fat-burning morning!

Before your patties are done, assemble your Avocado-Cucumber Spread. Cut into the ripe flesh of the avocado wedges right where you flipped the fish patties and scoop the fruit into the bowl with the cucumbers. Season with salt and a few grinds of pepper. Drizzle the organic extra-virgin olive oil over the mixture. Chop the avocados coarsely with your spatula. Discard any large avocado pieces. Taste for seasoning and adjust if needed. Plate the fish and avocados together. Dress the patties with the avocado-cucumber mixture. Toss the lettuce leaves in a light vinaigrette dressing, like our Champagne Vinaigrette, if desired, and wedge them between the avocado-cucumber spread and the top bun.

While your grill is preheating, prepare Avocado-Cucumber Spread. Put a Midori (or ice) melon baller to good use. When the grill is ready, clean the grill rack thoroughly and oil it to prevent the patties from sticking. Half an avocado lengthwise, remove the pit, and cut each half into thirds so you have 6 wedges per avocado. Using a spatula, transfer the patties to the grill. Arrange the avocado slices on the grill as well. With a brush, dress the avocados in avocado oil and grill for 1 minute per side. Rotate your fish patties 90 degrees at the halfway point for cross-hatch grill marks. Do not press the patties down with the edge of the spatula as they cook. This will squeeze the juices out of the meat and lead to starchiness. Instead, slip the blade beneath and gently lift the patties to rotate.

Preparation: Preheat your grill as high as it will go. Place the ginger-scallion salmon on a chopping board. Cut the slab into 1-inch chunks. Add the sesame and arrowroot. Pulse the fish into a mince. Scoop out about 1/6 of the fish paste and form a ball with your hands. Press the ball into a round patty. If your fingers stick to the fish, touch the patty lightly with a moistened hand. Form the patty slightly thinner than you'd like, about 1/2 inch thick, as it will plump up during grilling. Line a baking sheet with parchment paper and place the patties on it in a single layer. Season the patties with salt and brush with oil. Tip to avoid sticking: it's important to generously oil your patties, the grill grates, and the grill rack.

Garnishes: rosemary, top half (or 1/4 shallot, thinly sliced), 3-4 lettuce leaves.

Avocado-Cucumber Spread: 1 pound ripe avocados, 1 medium cucumber (about 3/4 pound), sea salt, freshly ground Tellicherry black pepper, 1-2 teaspoons organic extra-virgin olive oil.

Ingredients: Salmon Burger: 2 lbs Ginger-Scallion Salmon (crispy bite, will provide a burger with a slightly looser texture that is good for grilling), 1 lb omega-3-rich salmon fillet, 2 teaspoons sesame, 2 teaspoons arrowroot, sea salt, avocado oil.

The healthy fats in salmon and avocado make this a very satisfying meal that will keep you full and your body fueled throughout the night. Yields 6 servings of Salmon Burger with Avocado-Cucumber Spread.

Juicy Salmon Burgers with Avocado Cucumber Spread

CHAPTER 8

Snack Ideas

Buffalo Chicken Dip – Get ready to lose the chip bowl with this hot, cheesy dip made with tender chicken and tangy Buffalo sauce. This ultimate low carb comfort food is perfect for scooping veggies or cheese crisps. Recipe makes about 24, 2-tbsp servings at 1 carb each.

Italian Prosciutto-Wrapped Mozzarella Sticks – Restaurant quality appetizer at home! These sticks are easy to make but pack tons of flavor in every bite. Recipe makes 4 servings with 1 carb each.

Jalapeno Poppers – The perfect tailgate or game day snack, it doesn't get better than decadent bacon-wrapped jalapeno poppers. This ketogenic version has the perfect balance of heat and creaminess. Recipe makes 6 servings with 4 net carbs per serving.

Salted Caramel Gummies – Sweet and chewy, these tasty gummies are perfect for a quick and easy snack on the go. These taste just like salted caramels! Recipe makes 16 servings with 2 carbs each.

CHAPTER 9

Dessert Options

Italian Almond Macaroons: A keto perfect treat that's visually stunning, perfect tasting, and easy to make. It is also make ahead; you freeze the baked cookies in airtight containers, thaw and assemble them. Leading up to a wedding and special occasions, these low-carb Almond Macaroons are one of the dishes that I always make in advance. The entire recipe uses only 1 tsp of dried egg whites. If you find yourself not knowing what to do with the rest of the carton of advanced foods, ask your friends or community to pool together and buy that to make multiple double and triple batches of these Almond Macaroons. Please read the linked Introduction and blog post containing these "life lessons" before proceeding with these recipes. The reader can then choose simple vegan baking ingredients of these flavorful cookie essentials or the Wired Recipe Dried Egg Whites, the only exception to the years-long ingredient choice repeal. Understanding why 5 ingredients and no special baking skills are the life lesson I talked about these short cookies at length in the Essential Keto meal with...Whole-Food ingredient chapter.

Special occasions can be especially challenging for people following low-carbohydrate keto diets for optimal weight loss or blood sugar balance. That's because most celebratory desserts, including cookies, cakes, and pies, end up compromising the benefits of a high-fat, slow-burning keto meal. Listed below are eight flourless, sugar-free, delicious desserts.

CHAPTER 10

Beverages to Aid Weight Loss

Remember not to consume these keto drinks in great amounts. Your body may therefore be driven out by incredibly healthy drinks. This risk comes from drinks with a rich, high concentration of minerals, such as sodium and potassium, that can draw electrolytes from your cell. Your feeling of being dehydrated or malnourished may also be enhanced, and those are signs that can push you to cease taking these beverages immediately. Instead of ranging from one to the other, take a variety of drinks that will help you attain a good balance. Start with the basics, for instance, lemon water, and then advance onto the more complex beverages. Your keto drink's primary goal is to switch your carbohydrate level to fat so you can enter into a phase of fasting and lose weight. As a result, concentrate on the drinks that can allow you to maintain stable electrolyte levels, hydrate you, and allow you to maintain an even blood glucose than water can. At the same time, don't fail to remember the calorie meal you're getting from your liquid nourishment.

Chia Fresca - If you're new to keto drinks, let this be your stepping stone. This drink does an excellent job in your digestion system which makes an optimal keto drink.

Lemon Water - The best keto drink for many individuals is lemon water. Being thankful to both keto and water, eventually, you'll treasure both of them.

Some drinks are healthy, but some can easily lead you to gain unwanted weight. Beverages are easy to consume if you're trying to fuel up with extra phosphate and even more calories. However, if you're trying to shed some weight, it's wise to understand which drinks fall under the healthy category. If you're looking for delicious keto drinks other than water, you have a lot to choose from. However, these choices are perfectly suited for a keto diet and can help you reduce your weight. Sometimes, it takes a lot for someone to lose weight, but these keto drinks have offered a lot to many individuals. Here's a list of easy keto drinks that you can also enjoy.

CHAPTER 11

Tips for Successful Weight Loss

The black and white approach towards dieting is not providing long-term success for many. A healthy lifestyle should not feel punitive. It should be a permanent lifestyle change that supports your mental and physical well-being. Indulge in macaroni and cheese, cake, and wine over the course of a year, and use the rest of the year to eat well, exercise, and relax. Cut down on portion sizes, take leftovers home in a doggie bag, and split an appetizer the next time you dine out. Be kind to yourself and believe that what you are doing is finally going to make a difference. Concentrate on positive self-talk and love.

Some days you may feel frustrated that the weight isn't coming off as rapidly as you want. In order to lose body fat, your body must be in a caloric deficit. It takes a reduction of 3500-5000 weekly to produce 1 to 2 lbs of weight loss per week. 150 minutes of moderate exercise or 75 minutes of high intensity vigorous activity every week is needed to help support a healthy weight loss. Yes, I said it, exercise. This is the missing piece because in reality, anyone can lose weight by cutting their calorie intake. However, exercising is a great way to accelerate fat and calorie burn. The health benefits of exercise also help with sloth, depression, and myriad of disease states.

CHAPTER 12

Exercise and Keto Diet

Carb balancing with a ketogenic diet can support your training and help you perform better more often. You can get even more results by matching your level of carbs - or your fuel source - to your type, intensity and duration of workouts. Top acknowledges that "there are ways to 'train your body to burn fat' (i.e., to produce the necessary energy by breaking down body fat) even at a high training intensity level." These strategies support endurance athletes or those performing strenuous activities such as rock climbing and hiking. For other high-intensity efforts, however, you need to have some carbs in order to perform and to recover.

Not too long ago, fitness pros thought it was a good idea to tell you to go lift weights on a low-carb diet - and that you were making progress even if you were actually losing muscle mass. Thankfully, we've significantly upgraded our understanding of how food and exercise work together to optimize body composition. Now, evidence and research support the idea that you need the right nutrients in your body to both fuel your workouts and to recover from them. As Lori Top of Clean Plate Mama explains, "The right carbs in the right amounts at the right times will enable you to keep losing fat, build muscle and make strength gains - even on a low-carb diet."

CHAPTER 13

Tracking Your Progress

If there were a significant increase in the fasting blood sugar the following day, the entire situation would require more time to ask questions about your adherence to the plan and also adjustments regarding protein. You don't have to worry if the morning fasting blood sugar continues to drop on a daily basis once this approach has been adopted. Aim for numbers less than 85 to 90 for real success and record the entire process in your weekly journal; you may discover a pattern if results appear to plateau. Please note: Glycogen stores are restored when meals containing more than 100 grams of protein have been consumed during one of the standard high-protein days, and the subsequent fasting blood sugar will rise the following morning; this is more evident when protein builds 80% to 90% of calorie intake. Detect any mistakes that have been made before building your meals specifically for these days. Provide space in your journal for your results and feelings about the weekly changes encountered as well. When you address a column or two each day regarding how you have felt on the diet, you may refer to this information after the end of the initial phase of this 28-day fat loss plan.

You should track your fasting blood sugar in the morning while aiming for results of less than 85 to 90. Though not optimal, it does point out progress. In theory, since you're a fat-burner, your blood sugar should be lower on a ketosis plan compared to a standard low-carb plan, provided there's not a tremendous amount of protein consumed, which would automatically raise blood sugar. You can use daily fasting blood sugar levels as a means to identify which foods hinder your progress by causing an unwanted increase in the morning blood sugar results. If your morning fasting blood sugar is higher than it should be, you may compensate by eating low-carb vegetables without protein during the mid-afternoon or consuming a shake with just a single scoop of protein powder. It's safe to conclude that even during the high-protein days, your blood sugar still falls within the "safe" limits once the meal is consumed during the mid-afternoon, given that the protein is absent then. This method precludes the consumption of any protein for the remainder of the day.

CHAPTER 14

Overcoming Challenges

At the start of your keto meal plan, no matter how excited you might be to be following a diet that tastes good, you might still feel quite unwell. Don't be discouraged by the symptoms of "keto flu." Most people feel groggy, exhausted, foggy headed, or even jittery during the first week of the keto diet. Why? By dramatically (but healthfully) limiting the amount of sugar that you eat, you will deplete the amount of glycogen available in your cells. Your body, so used to the constant supply of simple-to-digest glucose, will have to summon some energy from fatty lipid stores instead. That requires a bit of an energy learning curve for the cells to adapt to. So it's only natural to feel slightly off. You may be left with the same symptoms as dehydration: brain fog, headaches, fatigue, and drowsiness. Not to worry. To chase away keto flu, hydrate often by sipping electrolyte- and mineral-rich drinks like bone broth, or eat water-rich veggies like cucumber, zucchini, and green leaf lettuce.

Now that you have been following a keto diet (and even if you haven't tried keto before), you will likely hit a few stumbling blocks along the way. Don't worry; it's normal. Life happens, especially when you're busy. And nothing is ever perfect (or else life would be so incredibly boring). In this section, I review some common obstacles that you might face when trying to lose weight on a keto meal plan, including known side effects of your new diet. Let's unravel the potential reasons why your body isn't doing what you want it to do, and we'll offer some solutions to help you through it, including "hacks" from the world of art. Okay, let's dig in.

CHAPTER 15

Frequently Asked Questions

No, that's "ketoacidosis" (a potentially life-threatening situation that is altogether different from "nutritional ketosis"). "Cessation," as many of us in this low-carb and ketogenic community will often refer to it, is rarely experienced in individuals properly operating on their delicate internal balance of macronutrients. Rather, it's the other way around! Ketosis is regularly sought out and happily sustained by health-minded individuals who realize the many benefits accompanied by this fat-burning metabolic state.

I thought ketosis was bad! Don't you get sick and die from it?

It sure does, but it's not! And you're not alone in questioning this crazy ketogenic concept at first. So many of us have spent a good portion of our lives not just dodging the dreaded "f" word, but sincerely striving to avoid it (along with a host of other "forbidden" foods and nutrients I discuss in greater detail earlier in the book under the heading "Nutrition Myths and Dogma"). The point is, much of what we've been traditionally programmed to believe about dietary fat is just plain wrong! Years of research have now supported what countless fat-torching individuals will also testify to: consuming a predominantly fat-fueled diet is indeed a method for OCR—for losing body fat and not just some of it, but an impressive amount of it—at that.

I can eat fat and lose fat, for real? It sounds like such an oxymoron.

CHAPTER 16

Conclusion

Next, we gave you a guide to getting your kitchen ready for the strictest keto plan achievable. Everything you've cooked since has been touched and changed by your hard work and new-to-you gadgets. Consistency is crucial for keto diets. If you can do this every day, uninterrupted, you could see your palate change, shedding the salty, oily foods for delicacies you've never even tried. Remember, fat loss is not simply about you eating fewer carbohydrates than you burn in an average day. Additionally, you may eat bigger, more filling meals, which recent studies have proven to be even better for Panzera Ks. Eating just 2 meals daily has its health risks as well and isn't good for you. Furthermore, although we discussed distractions, you may experience a wide range of goals and needs (fine dining experiences, in-between meal snacks, different nutritional makeup, etc.) Thus, it's important to balance out your new way of life and appropriately measure to assure your success. Consider supplementing any food urgencies with Chrissy Doyle's latest book, 15-Minute Keen (Fat Burning) Compensations.

We started Fat-Burning Feast: Keto Meals for Optimal Weight Loss by telling you that the hardest part of any diet is sticking to it and ensuring that the diet you follow includes keto-friendly foods. You probably thought it was about the recipes, but in the end, it's the ingredients that go into making life-altering recipes. If we've done our job right, you've been eating some of the best keto diet-approved foods. And if we've done our job even marginally well, you've found your new normal and banked the food emergency funds you've needed to sustain the new you. You've just maximized your chances for success and recovery on the fly.

Milton Keynes UK
Ingram Content Group UK Ltd.
UKHW040938081224
452111UK00011B/229